The Flower
Savannah, GA.
31401

I0513491

YOUNG BILLY'S HANDS IS ALL COVERED WITH GERMS

(HE NEVER USED SOAP)

The Flower
COPYRIGHT 2018

YOUNG BILLY'S HANDS IS ALL COVERED WITH GERMS

(HE NEVER USED SOAP)

(WRITE BY)\

"THE FLOWER"

DEDICATION

THIS DEDICATION IS TO MY FAMILY AND A SPECIAL FRIEND

TABLE OF CONTENTS

WHAT HE LOVED

Insects and animals	7
Dinner	13
Looking for more	14
Bitten	15
Bumps grew	18
Hospitalized	20
Washing hands	24

Billy loves to play with animals, insect, dirt, climb trees but he would never thoroughly wash his hands. He would dig in the sand, playing with all sought of things and half wash his hands.

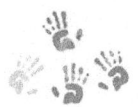

He loved to dig for worms, and stretch them out sometimes with juice oozing from their bodies. He would play with them for hours putting them on tree limbs but afterwards, he would rinse his hands off with water

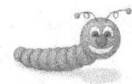

He would hunt for beetles; he loved the big one with the red and black color. He sometimes let them crawl all over his hands, at then he collected them up and put them into jars, but afterwards, he would rinse his hands off with water.

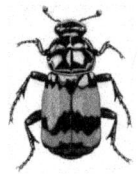

He takes all his dump trucks outside, when he goes to play. He'll roll them in the dirt and mud, sometimes they'll be cover all over with mud, but afterwards, he would rinse his hands off with water.

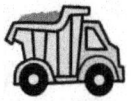

He loved to climb trees, he would see the butterfly cocoons and pull them down, so that he could take one home. He wanted to see how they change into a butterfly, but afterwards, he would rinse his hands off with water.

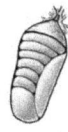

He also loved to go to the pond, to catch and play with the frogs and their Lilly pads. Sometimes he picks them up and they would leave a trial of slim on his hands, but afterwards, he would just rinse his hands off with water.

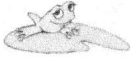

Next, he looks for snails and finds a nest of them. He picks a few of them up and let them crawl around in his hands over and over again, after he puts them down, he rinses his hands off with just plain water.

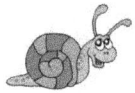

Every day when his mom calls him in to eat his dinner, she would tell him to get clean up before he eats. He goes in the bathroom and rinses his hands off with water, never washing them with soap. He sits down and eats his dinner, afterwards he goes back outside to play.

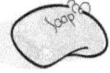

Next he searches through the grass, trying to catch a few lizards to put in his jar. He loves to see them change colors and also show their blankets, but afterwards he would rinse his hands off with water, never using any soap.

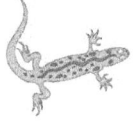

When he goes outside to play with his friends, he digs in the dirt hoping to find some fire ants to add to his collection, but while he sits with his hand on the ground, he is bitten by a few ants, so he goes inside and rinses his hands off, never using any soap. He never told his parents he was bitten by fire ants

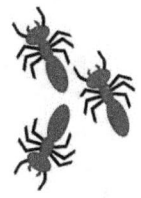

Later, his head begins to spin, so he goes to take a bath, never cleaning his hands with soap. He lies down and goes to sleep but when he wakes up the small bumps on his hand had spread and gotten larger.

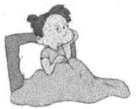

He begins wearing long sleeve shirts to hide the bumps when he goes out to play and when he hunt for insects, afterwards when he goes inside, he rinses his hands off never using soap.

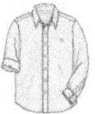

The bumps on him grew larger and begin to spread more and more up his arm, it was completely covered. They begin to itch all the time, he scratched in school, at home, but especially at the dinner table. It got so bad, that he accidently knocked over the table with all the food on it.

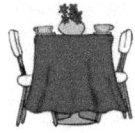

Billy's parents noticed his constant scratching, and took him into the bathroom to see what was wrong. When they took off his shirt, they nearly pasted out from the way his arm looked. They rushed him to the doctor's office, so that he can take a look at his arm.

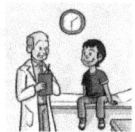

The doctor was shock at the site of it and admitted him in the hospital. He was given medication to help him get better. The doctor found out that he had been bitten by fire ants, and because he didn't properly wash his hands made it worse.

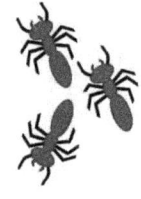

Billy didn't wash nor scrubbed his hands with soap, that made the germs spread onto the bumps, so The more he scratched them the worse it got. Scratching caused the bumps to get infected and spread up his arm.

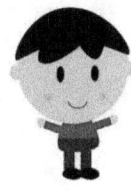

Billy stayed in the hospital for two weeks and the doctor explains to him, how important hand washing is. It was a close call because he almost lost his arm due to germs and bacteria.

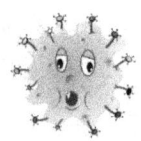

After Billy was release from the hospital, he asks his mom to buy him lots of soap. Now when he goes outside to hunt for insect he grabs the soap and washes his hands; at lease now, he makes sure to keep his hands clean and germ free.

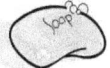

Practice good hand washing, it keeps your hands germ free and you won't end up like Billy. Always scrub under your finger nails and use lot of soap to keep your hands clean. Even keep hand sanitizer to help out.

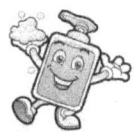

(END)

BIOGRAPHY

Ms. D. Mae Ward use to work around children for twenty years, they would tell her what books they like to read, this inspired her to write fictional short stories. She is a member of the blue moon and poetry club. She lives with her family in Georgia. She loves to write music, poetry and travel in her spare time.

www.ingramcontent.com/pod-product-compliance
Lightning Source LLC
Chambersburg PA
CBHW062238220526
45471CB00009B/3529